Ingredients of a Balanced Diet

Fruits

Rachel Eugster

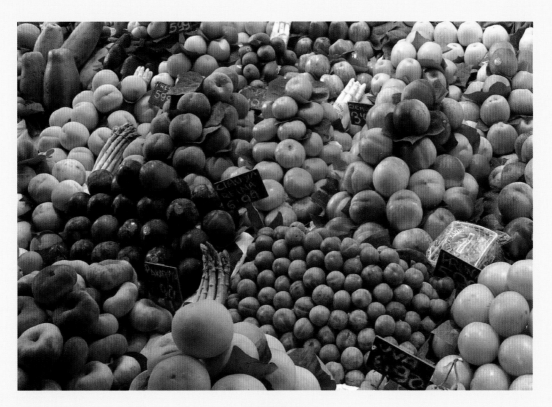

FRANKLIN
WATTS

First published in 2007 by
Franklin Watts
338 Euston Road,
London NW1 3BH

Franklin Watts Australia
Hachette Children's Books
Level 17/207 Kent Street
Sydney NSW 2000

INGREDIENTS OF A BALANCED DIET:
FRUITS was produced for Franklin Watts by
Bender Richardson White, PO Box 266,
Uxbridge, UK.
Editor and Picture Researcher: Lionel Bender
Designer and Page Make-up: Ben White
Cover Make-up: Mike Pilley, Radius
Production: Kim Richardson
Graphics and Maps: Stefan Chabluk

A CIP catalogue record for this book is
available from the British Library.

ISBN: 978 0 7496 6804 4
Dewey classification: 641.3'4

Printed in China

Note to parents and teachers: Every effort has
been made by the Publishers to ensure that the
websites in this book are suitable for children,
that they are of the highest educational value,
and that they contain no inappropriate or
offensive material. However, because of the
nature of the Internet, it is impossible to
guarantee that the contents of these sites will
not be altered. We strongly advise that Internet
access is supervised by a responsible adult.

Franklin Watts is a division of Hachette
Children's Books

Picture credits

Cover image: FoodandDrinks agency.
foodanddrinkphotos.com: pages 4, 7 top, 9, 10
(Graham Ainsley), 11, 17, 22, 27. iStockphotos:
pages 1, 3 and all Food bite panels (Heidi Tuller);
pages 1 and 5 (Sophie Gist); 3 and 16 (Ursula
Alter); 7 right (Anssi Ruuska); repeated image on
Recipe panels (Jim Jurica); 12 (Marek Tihelka); 14
(Tatiana Sayig); 15 (Kelly Kline); 18; 19 (Joszef
Szazy-Fabian); 20 (Roberto Lorente); 21 (Will
Rennick); 23 (Olga Shelego); 24 (Gert Very); 26
(Ronnie Comeau); 30, 31, 32 (Edyta Pawlowska).
Cover image: foodanddrinkphotos.com.
BRW wishes to thank Sarah Bell and colleagues at
foodanddrinkphotos.com for setting up the
commissioned photography.

The author

Rachel Eugster is a food, health and
nutrition writer and editor. Formerly food
editor of *Walking* magazine, she is a
regular contributor to *Continental* and *Yes
Mag* and creates recipes for people of all
ages. She feeds her family as healthy a diet
as they will eat!

The consultant

Ester Davies is a professional food and
nutrition writer, lecturer and consultant.
She has a B.Ed. in Food, Nutrition and
Sociology. She has written books on food
specifically for the National Curriculum.

Note: In recipes, liquid measures and
small quantities are given by volume in
millilitres (ml) as this is how measuring
jugs and spoons are usually marked.

Contents

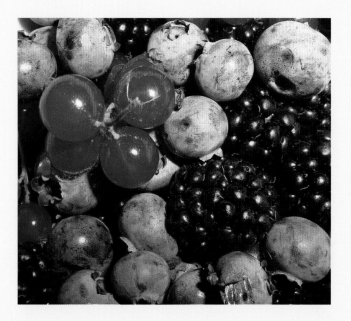

Major nutrients

Sugars and starches, or carbohydrates: give you energy. Fibre, or roughage, is a kind of carbohydrate that helps digestion. Many fruits are rich in carbohydrates.

Proteins: provide building materials for bones, hair, muscles and skin. Fruits are low in proteins.

Vitamins and minerals: help you fight disease, digest food and strengthen your bones and teeth. Fruits are good sources of these.

Fats: store energy and carry vitamins to where they are needed. Fats from plant foods (unsaturated fats) are better for you than those from meat and dairy products (saturated fats).

Food for life

Fruits are the parts of flowering plants that contain the seeds. There are many kinds of fruits, from citrus fruits (for example oranges, grapefruits, lemons and tangerines), grapes and melons (for instance honeydew and canteloupe) to berries, apples, blackcurrants, pears and pineapples.

We even eat some fruits as vegetables – for example tomatoes, aubergines and cucumbers. Pods containing beans, peas or lentils are fruits. We eat them fresh as vegetables or dried as pulses. Nuts are dry fruits with a hard shell.

In this book, we look at how and why fruits should be part of your diet. Doctors and nutritionists, or food scientists, recommend that you eat at least five portions of fruits and vegetables a day, along with water, grains, proteins and certain fats, and very little sugar and salt.

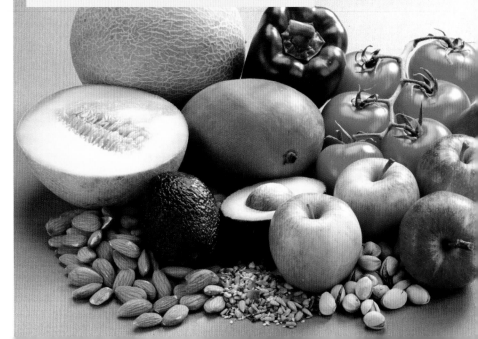

▼ Fruits – and the seeds they contain – come in many shapes, sizes and forms.

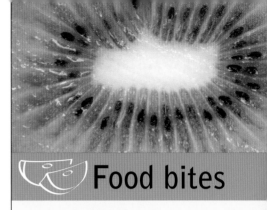

Choosing the right foods

For your diet, 'balanced' means just the right amounts and different types of foods. Eating a wide variety of good foods, exercising and avoiding bad foods is the key to being healthy and fit.

Foods and drinks contain various nutrients (see panel on page 4), which are materials your body needs but cannot make itself. Nutrients allow your body to work properly, to stay healthy and active, and to grow. The types of nutrients you need, and how much, depend on your age and size, whether you are a boy or girl, how active you are and how fast you are growing.

Energy

Foods and drinks contain energy, too. You need energy for all activity – to make your muscles work, and for thinking, breathing and digesting. Energy in foods and drinks is measured in kilocalories (kcal) or kilojoules (kJ). One kilocalorie equals 4.2 kilojoules. A balanced diet gives you just the right number of kilocalories. You will need more kilocalories when you are active and playing sport than when you are studying, reading or sleeping. Energy you do not use is stored as fat.

Food bites

Fruit servings

One serving of fruit is about the same size as the palm of your hand. This is equivalent to:

2 or more small fruits:
(2 kiwis, 2 apricots, 2 plums, 14 cherries)
1 medium fruit: (1 apple, pear, banana, orange)
1 slice large fruit: (melon, pineapple, papaya)
1/2 a whole large fruit: (grapefruit)
about 50g to 100g dried fruit: (apricots, figs, dates)
1 medium glass fruit juice: but even 100% pure juice counts only once per day because it has very little fibre.

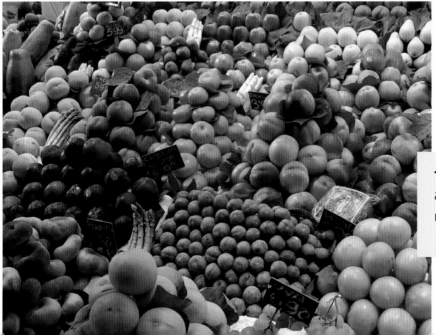

◀ At a food market, you will find a variety of fruits. Eat as wide a range of fruits as you can.

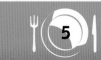

Food groups and diet

Foods are often sorted into groups based on the nutrients they provide. Most nutritionists group foods into five categories. To help you know what and how much to eat from any group, nutritionists have created diagrams like those shown below. In the food pyramid, fruits are placed on the lowest level. This means you can eat lots of them. Some versions of this diagram place plant oils at the bottom and butter and lard at the top to remind you to include some unsaturated fat in your diet but to limit saturated fat.

Food pyramid and food plate

A food pyramid: Eat lots from the bottom layer – which includes fruits – and less from the top layer.

A food plate: One quarter is protein-rich and the rest is a mix of vegetables, fruits and grains.

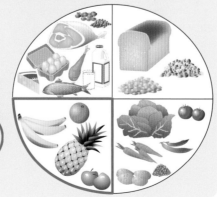

Nutrition facts

Main food groups

1. **Bread, other grain products, and potatoes:** These are rich in carbohydrates (including fibre) and are good sources of proteins, minerals and vitamins.
2. **Fruits and vegetables:** These are rich in carbohydrates (including fibre), vitamins and minerals.
3. **Red meat, poultry, seafood, eggs, nuts, seeds and pulses:** These are good sources of proteins, minerals and B vitamins but may also contain saturated fats.
4. **Milk and dairy products:** These are good sources of calcium and proteins.
5. **Fatty, sugary and salty foods:** These contain a mix of nutrients but also unwanted fats, calories and salt.

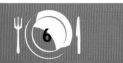

▼ Add fruit to your meals. This dinner includes turkey in a creamy sauce with avocado strips and orange segments, served with a tropical fruit juice.

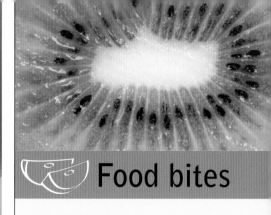

Food bites

Water

About two-thirds of your body weight is water. To stay healthy, your body needs about two litres of water a day – a litre from the foods you eat and a litre from what you drink. Fruits and fruit juices can provide much of this, but you should drink some plain water, too.

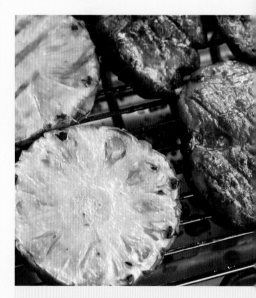

▲ Eating fruit such as pineapple with meat will give you a wide range of nutrients.

Fruits alongside other foods

One way to eat a balanced diet is to imagine that your plate is divided into four equal sections. Fill one quarter with protein-rich foods such as beef or lamb (red meats), poultry (white meat), dairy products, fish, nuts or pulses. Fill the other three quarters with fruits, vegetables, brown rice, potatoes, bread or pasta – any foods from the bottom layer of the food pyramid. This small change can make a big difference in your diet.

Eating fruits is essential for good health. You probably do not eat as much fruit as you should. To be certain of getting all the nutrients you need, try to eat some fruit at every meal.

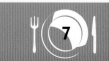

Inside fruits

Fruits should make up one-third of your diet. They provide many vitamins (for details see page 22) and some minerals, as shown in the panel on the right. Fruits also contain various chemicals that give them their colours and flavours and are good for you.

Fruits also offer quick energy, in the form of natural sugars, and even some proteins. They are high in fibre, which helps digestion. Some prepared fruits, however, contain fat, salt and refined sugar, so it is better to eat fresh fruit, if you can.

Nutrition facts

Different types of fruits – with their seeds

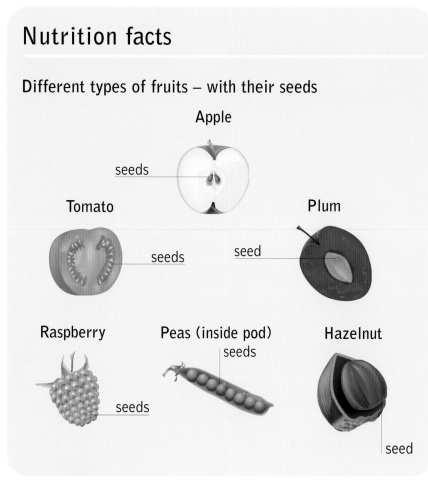

Apple

seeds

Tomato

Plum

seeds

seed

Raspberry

Peas (inside pod)

Hazelnut

seeds

seeds

seed

Nutrition facts

Minerals in fruits

Calcium
This is needed for healthy teeth and bones.

Iron
Red blood cells need iron to carry oxygen round the body.

Phosphorus
Phosphorus helps the release and use of energy in foods.

Magnesium
This is needed for many chemical reactions in the body.

Sodium and chloride
Together, these control water balance in the body. Sodium is needed for healthy muscles and nerves.

Apricots, prunes, figs and dates are excellent fruit sources of minerals.

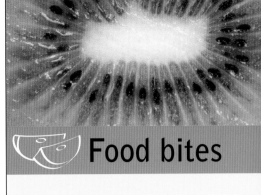

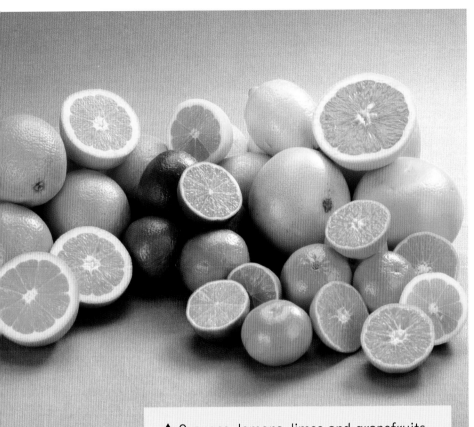

▲ Oranges, lemons, limes and grapefruits are popular citrus fruits. Each has a thick skin and a fleshy, juicy inside.

Pectin

Fibre is found only in plant foods. It comes in two forms, namely soluble and insoluble. Pectin is the main soluble fibre in fruits. During digestion, it partly dissolves into a jelly-like substance that removes toxins, which are possibly harmful chemicals in foods. Pectin is present in the skin and flesh of many fruits. Apples are a particularly good source.

Insoluble fibre passes through your body largely unchanged. It helps your body move out the parts of food that it cannot use, just the way a broom sweeps out rubbish. Getting rid of undigested food keeps your digestive system in good working order. Fruit skins are a good source of insoluble fibre.

Citrus fruits

Lemons, oranges, limes, tangerines, grapefruits and kumquats are known as citrus fruits because they contain lots of citric acid, which has a sour taste.

Citrus fruits are rich in vitamin C, which your body cannot make.

A lack of vitamin C causes scurvy, a disease that results in bleeding from small blood vessels and the gums.

Most citrus fruits originally came from China, India and South-east Asia. Today, the major citrus fruit-growing regions are Florida and California in North America, the Mediterranean region, South Africa and Central America.

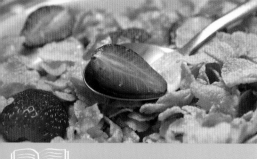

Recipe

Fruit rainbows

Makes 4 servings.

Ingredients

175g raspberries or halved
  strawberries
1 peach or 2 apricots, sliced
1 banana, sliced
1 kiwi or 5 green grapes, halved
125g blueberries or blackberries
240ml natural yogurt

Preparation

On each of four plates, spread one-
  quarter of the yogurt to make a
  'cloudy sky'. You can use
  blueberry yogurt if you want a
  dark sky.
Arrange the fruits in arcs on top
  of the yogurt to look like a
  rainbow.

Rainbow Smoothie Variation:
Purée the fruits and yogurt in a
blender or food processor with a
little sugar to taste and a little
ice. Pour the smoothie into
glasses and serve.

▶ Sharing this bowl of fruit
and drinking a glass of juice
will give each of these
children two or three servings
of fruit.

The fruits you eat now

Perhaps the most important thing that fruits do for you is to fight disease. Eating fruits every day can help you avoid heart disease, stroke, cancer and diabetes. It can also help keep your digestive system and your eyes, bones and teeth healthy, and help reduce the effects of ageing.

Below average

Most Europeans and North Americans eat less fruits and vegetables than they should. The average European eats fewer than three servings a day, and the average American only a little over three servings. Children eat even less than these adult average amounts. This may not cause harm, but it makes balancing a diet with a proper range of nutrients difficult. You should try and increase the amount of fruit you eat.

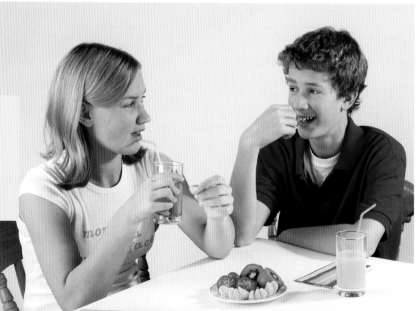

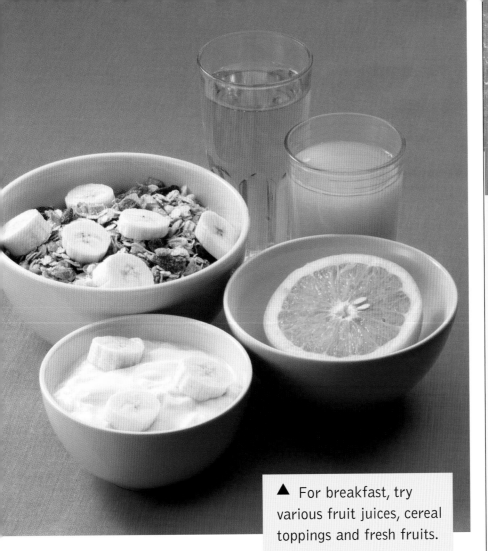

▲ For breakfast, try various fruit juices, cereal toppings and fresh fruits.

Energy versus nutrients

Maybe you drink fruit juice most mornings, along with half a grapefruit or an orange? Perhaps you have fresh or dried fruit with your breakfast cereal? You might also have a piece of fruit with lunch or for a snack. You certainly eat a little fruit in pies, cakes and even sometimes in biscuits.

While biscuits and cakes make nice treats, you should not eat large quantities of them. They usually have a lot of saturated fat and sugars added to them. They contain many 'empty calories' – energy-giving substances in food that are not combined with any essential nutrients. Also, any fruit is usually present in only tiny amounts.

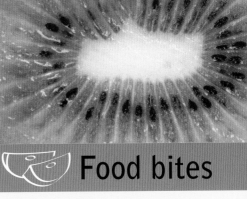

Food bites

Go for fruit not fizz

One way to a healthier diet is to drink 100% juice or fruit smoothies instead of fizzy drinks. Most fizzy drinks have lots of sugar or artificial sweeteners and only a little fruit. If you stop drinking fizzy drinks for a while, you might even find that when you taste them again you don't like them very much. Do drink lots of plain water, too. Too much fruit juice can lead to tooth decay.

Think big

The largest edible fruit is the pumpkin. Giant pumpkins weigh more than 650kg – about 20 times your weight. Grapefruits grow to 3kg, apples to 1.7kg, pineapples to 8kg and strawberries to 240g.

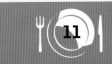

From fresh to dried

Fruits are everywhere. As well as fresh fruits, tinned and frozen fruits are available. There are also dried fruits, for example raisins, figs and dates. Fruits are dried by placing them in direct sunlight, heating them in ovens or removing the moisture in them using an electric machine called a dehydrator. Fruits are healthy to eat fresh, frozen or dried.

An expanding range

In earlier times, available fruits were limited to those that grew nearby or were in season. Nowadays, fruits are flown from faraway places to markets all over the world. Fruits that were once known only where they grow are now widespread, such as coconuts, mangoes, kiwis and papayas. Farmers are also creating new varieties of fruits and these are quickly introduced into shops.

Nutrition facts

Extra benefits

Some of the colours and flavours in fruits have been found to be as important to our health as vitamins. These chemicals lose some of their effectiveness once the fruits have ripened and during storage. The more different kinds of fruits you eat, from fresh apples and pears to dried apricots, figs and dates, the better the mix of these nutrients you will get.

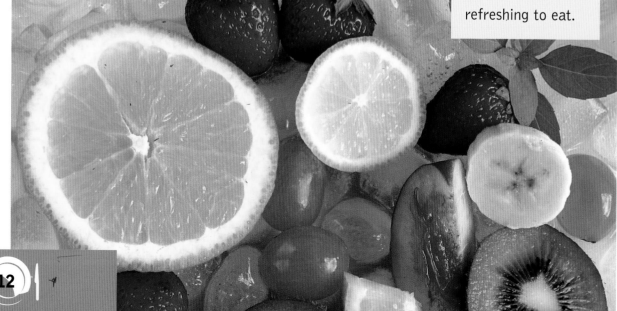

▼ Chilled fruits are refreshing to eat.

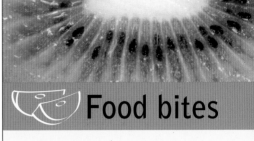

Ideal food packages

Fruits are good for many reasons. You can eat them just as they are with no preparation necessary beyond washing or peeling. Most fruits fit perfectly in your hand so are easy to carry and to eat while you are on the move. Because fruits generally contain few calories and little or no fats or refined sugars, you can eat as much as you like as part of a balanced diet.

An unusual way to eat more fruit is to try frozen fruit as an alternative to fruit salad, ice lollies and ice cream. Thread grapes and slices of oranges, kiwis, melons, peaches and bananas on to skewers and put them in a freezer until hard.

Where in the world?

The fruits you eat come mainly from three main climate zones.

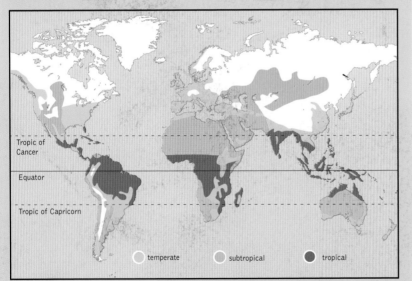

Tropic of Cancer

Equator

Tropic of Capricorn

○ temperate   ○ subtropical   ● tropical

TEMPERATE
plums, apples, peaches, pears, strawberries, tomatoes

SUBTROPICAL
oranges, lemons, grapefruits, avocados, figs, olives

TROPICAL
bananas, pineapples, coconuts, mangoes, star fruits, guavas, melons

Food bites

Which type to buy?

There is no bad way to eat fruit, but each type you buy has its own set of advantages.

Fresh fruit
- best taste, texture and look
- high in fibre and nutrients, especially when ripe
- often cheap in season
- you can sometimes pick your own from the plants.

Dried fruit
- particularly high in fibre
- high in calories if you need lots of energy for hard work
- available off-season
- can be easily stored.

Frozen or tinned
- can be better than fresh if frozen at peak ripeness
- available off-season
- can be easily stored.
Do, though, avoid tinned fruits in syrups as they are very sugar-rich.

Meals with fruits

Any healthy food you eat replaces some unhealthy food in your diet and provides better nutrients. Here are some tasty ways to eat more fruit.

Breakfast

Fruit is a familiar breakfast food, especially drunk as juice. You can upgrade juice into a 'smoothie' by blending it with low-fat yogurt and fresh or frozen fruit.

Dried fruit (such as raisins, dates, cranberries, cherries) and fresh fruit are great additions to cold cereals and porridge. You can make toppings for toast, pancakes or waffles by cooking fruits such as raspberries, apricots or plums with a little honey, and then puréeing in a blender or food processor.

▼ Pancakes are delicious with berries or a fruit syrup made with honey.

Nutrition facts

Bananarama

Bananas offer minerals and fibre, some vitamins and even a little protein. Here are some more interesting banana facts.

- Bananas are the fourth leading crop in the world (after rice, maize and wheat).
- Bananas grow upside-down from one of the world's largest bunches of flowers.
- Only 15% of the bananas grown worldwide are sweet fruit. The rest – plantain bananas – are eaten as a staple food, which means that they are a basic part of the diet, eaten like rice, bread or potatoes might be elsewhere.
- One banana gives you enough energy for 26 minutes of cycling.

Grapes and other fruits go well with cheeses as a dessert.

Lunch and dinner

Fresh apples, pears, bananas, nectarines, plums and chunks of melon can be eaten with or between meals. Dried fruits also make good snacks. Try figs, apricots, mango chunks, papaya slices, apples, peaches and pears. You can also mix dried fruit with nuts and seeds.

Slices of apples, oranges, tangerines and avocados are great for lunchtime salads. For dinner dishes, the flavours of fruits balance well with many meats, for example oranges with duck, apples with pork, lemons or cranberries with chicken and turkey. Dried fruit can liven up an otherwise plain grain dish.

What is for dessert?

In desserts, fruit can play a starring role. It appears in many bakery goods, such as flans, tarts and pies – but so do saturated fats and sugars. Fruit can be enjoyed fresh on its own, or stewed – as compote – and topped with low-fat yogurt or ice cream. Melted chocolate and toffee are good dipping sauces for fresh fruits such as strawberries, or apple and banana chunks. Pieces of frozen fruit are mouth-watering (see page 12).

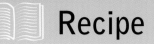

Recipe

Cranberry-orange sunburst turkey

Makes 6 servings.
Ingredients
350g cranberries, fresh or frozen
1 large onion, sliced
1 skinless, boneless turkey breast (about 1 kg)
375ml orange juice, thick with pulp
80ml olive oil
100g sugar
120ml balsamic vinegar
5ml rosemary
2.5ml pepper

Preparation
Preheat the oven to 200°C (Gas mark 6). Put the onions and cranberries into a shallow baking dish. Place the turkey breast on top. Combine the remaining ingredients and pour them over the turkey.

Roast the breast for an hour, basting it occasionally. Before you remove it from the oven, check the meat is cooked right through by cutting into it a little with a knife. If it is not, continue for another 10 minutes until cooked.

Serve slices of the turkey, with its sauce, with rice, couscous, bulgur or quinoa.

Warm, easy-zap jams

Makes 240ml each.
Ingredients
150g sliced strawberries
100g sugar
5ml lemon juice
 OR
150g blueberries
100g sugar
1.2ml cinnamon

Preparation
Combine the ingredients in a very
 large, microwave-safe bowl.
 Microwave on high power for
 4 minutes.
Stir the mixture well. Microwave
 for another 2 to 6 minutes until
 the mixture is thicker and has
 boiled for at least 1 full minute.
Allow the hot liquid to cool for
 about 10 minutes then stir and
 serve warm with pancakes or
 scones.

▶Berries are ideal for puréeing
to make a smoothie. Wash them
first, as you should any fruit, to
remove any dirt and pesticides.

Making fruits last

Fresh fruit should be washed in cool water to remove any dirt, pesticides and microorganisms. These are removed naturally from fruits that you peel to eat, for example oranges. Whether you remove the skin of fruits such as apples and pears is a matter of taste, but the skin is a good source of fibre.

Firm fruits should be scrubbed with a clean brush when possible. This is particularly important with melons, as slicing them can transfer bacteria from their rinds to the inside of the fruit.

Take care not to knock soft fruits, as once their peel or skin is damaged they may spoil more quickly.

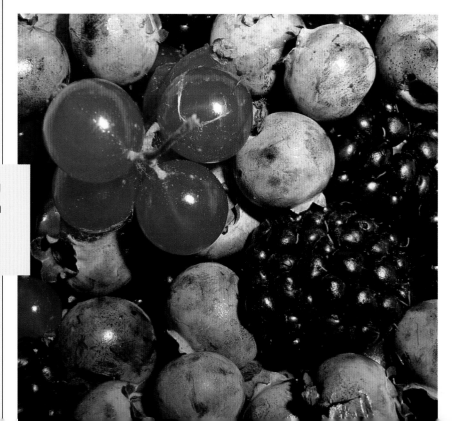

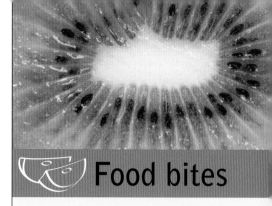

Storage

Fruits that ripen fast, such as berries and peaches, should be kept in a refrigerator, preferably in a plastic drawer. Cut fruits should also be kept in the refrigerator. Be sure that fish and meat are stored below other foods so their juices cannot drip on any fruits (or vegetables) you may want to eat raw.

Many fruits can be kept at room temperature. To maintain quality or speed up ripening, fruits such as bananas, tomatoes and pears, are best kept in a cool, dry place. Mouldy, shrivelled or slimy fruit should be thrown away.

Fruits can be preserved for months by drying or by heating and sealing them in jars or tins from which air is removed. These products are often called 'preserves'.

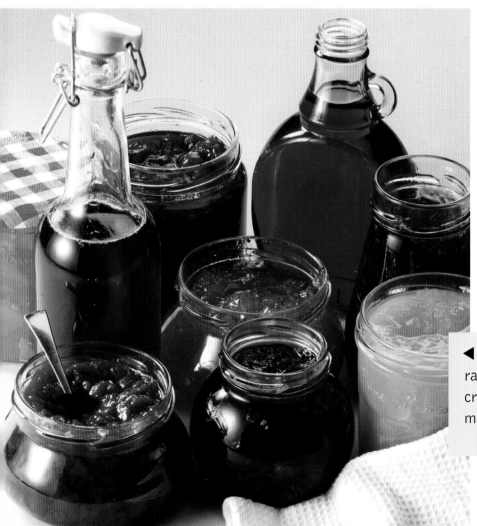

Food bites

Fruit preparations

These are some ways fruits are used or served. Can you think of others?

Compote Fruit that has been cooked slowly with sugar or syrup.

Jam Fruit that has been boiled with sugar until the mixture sets.

Jelly This is made like jam but with the juice not the flesh of the fruit.

Liquor The liquid in which fruit has been cooked. It has taken some of the flavour, colour and nutrients from the fruit.

Syrup A liquid created by dissolving sugar in hot water or fruit juice.

◀ Fruits such as oranges, lemons, raspberries, strawberries and cranberries are preserved as jams, marmalades, jellies and syrups.

Tropical lamb skewers

Makes 4 servings.
Ingredients
500g lamb, cubed (about 16
  pieces)
2 star fruits
12 kumquats
juice of 1 lemon (about 60ml)
60ml honey
15ml olive oil
4 skewers, metal or wood (first
  soaked in water)

Preparation
The night before, in a bowl, mix
  the honey, lemon juice and olive
  oil. Add the lamb cubes, mix
  well, and leave to marinate
  overnight in the refrigerator.
Cut each star fruit into four slices.
  Using your fingers, and
  alternating the items, push four
  pieces of lamb, three kumquats
  and two slices of star fruits on
  to each skewer.
Grill the skewers (turning them
  over once or twice) until the
  lamb is cooked. This will take
  about 5 to 8 minutes each side.

Traditional fruit diets

Because most plants produce fruits naturally, our ancestors did not need to invest any energy in growing or preparing them. Today, there are several traditional fruit-based diets that are recognised as being particularly healthy.

Latin American and Mediterranean diets

The traditional Latin American diet is based on fresh fruits, beans, grains, tubers, nuts and vegetables. The fruits include bananas, mangoes, pineapples and citrus fruits. The Mediterranean diet – especially in Italy and Greece – is built around a single fruit: the olive. Olives are eaten on their own as appetisers, in salads and in cooked dishes. Olive oil is the principal source of fat.

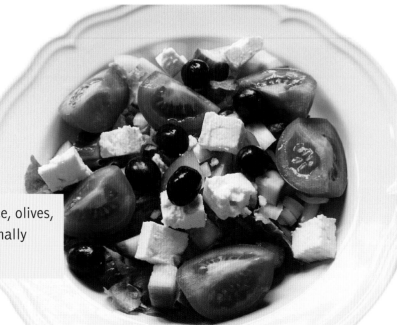

▶Greek salad, with cucumber, lettuce, olives, tomatoes and feta (a cheese traditionally made from sheep's or goat's milk).

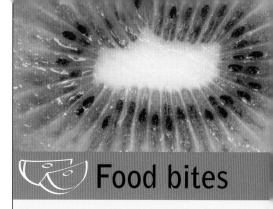

People in olive-growing regions use olive oil in much the same way others use butter. They cook with it, use it in salad dressings and even dip their bread into it.

From grapes and dried fruits to coconuts

In Greece, Turkey and neighbouring countries, people eat lots of grapes, nuts, figs, tomatoes and aubergines. These may be eaten as snacks or used in salads and cooked dishes. Cheese, yogurt, fish and poultry are often eaten, but red meat is eaten only a few times a month. Fruit is the typical daily dessert. Most sweet dishes are sweetened with honey rather than sugar. In the Middle East, fresh and dried fruits are often eaten as snacks and are used widely in cooked dishes.

Fruits have also been staple foods in many places throughout history. Examples include durians in Southeast Asia, avocados in Mexico, coconuts throughout the tropics, jackfruit and breadfruit in the tropical Pacific islands and plantains in East Africa.

Dried fruits

Since the first civilisations 5,000 years ago, people have dried fruits to eat. Dried fruits need no further preparation before they are eaten or used in cooking. They include:

Apples cut into segments or rings

Apricots as whole fruits

Berries for example blueberries and cranberries, as whole fruits

Dates as whole fruits

Figs as whole fruits

Grapes seedless varieties, in the form of raisins and sultanas

Peaches and nectarines as halves or segments

Plums as whole fruits, in the form of prunes

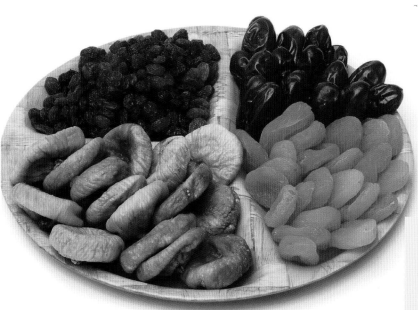

◀ Popular dried fruits include dates, figs, apricots and sultanas. These are often eaten on their own as appetizers or snacks.

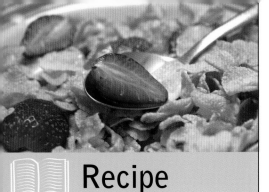

Recipe

Fruit explosion curry

Makes 6 servings.

Ingredients

15ml olive oil

1 onion, chopped

175g fresh pumpkin, cut into bite-
sized chunks

190g rice

75g hazelnuts, coarsely chopped

30ml curry powder

2 apples

40g raisins

125ml apple juice

480ml water

toppings: bananas, mangoes and
pineapples cut into bite-sized
chunks; grated unsweetened
coconut; low-fat yogurt; chutney.

Preparation

Preheat oven to 190°C (Gas mark
5). Heat the oil in a heavy, oven-
proof pan. Add the onion and
sauté (fry) for 2 minutes.

Add the pumpkin and sauté for 2
minutes. Add the rice, hazelnuts
and curry; stir and heat through.

Add the apples, raisins, apple juice
and water. Cover the pan and
bring to a boil.

Stir the mixture once and transfer
the pan to the oven. Bake for
about 25 minutes, stirring once
or twice, until the liquid is
absorbed and the rice is tender.

Add your choice of toppings.

Vegetarians and vegans

A vegetarian is someone who does not eat meat, including red meat such as lamb and beef, fish or white meat from poultry such as chicken and turkey. Vegans are people who eat no animal foods at all – meat, fish, shellfish, eggs, cheese or milk.

Some people are vegetarians or vegans by choice. The followers of the religions Hinduism and Buddhism do not eat meat as they usually believe no harm should be done to animals. People in poor parts of the world have no choice – they may not be able to buy meat or none is available for long periods.

▼ Avocados are high in protein, fibre, B vitamins, folic acid, zinc and healthy fats. Avocados can be made into dips (such as guacamole), and added to salads.

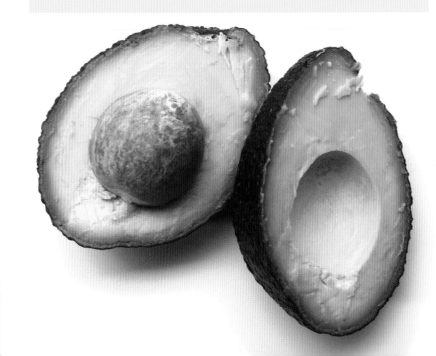

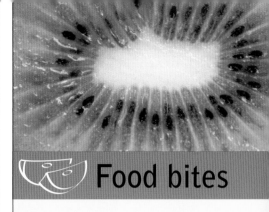

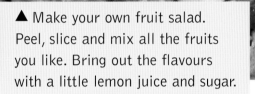

▲ Make your own fruit salad. Peel, slice and mix all the fruits you like. Bring out the flavours with a little lemon juice and sugar.

How fruit can help

Meat, fish and dairy products are the main sources of protein and many vitamins and minerals. If you are not eating these foods, you should eat a range of foods to help balance your diet. Although most fruits are not a major source of proteins, some fruits – especially avocados, guavas and coconuts – are rich in them. Dried figs are rich in the minerals iron and calcium, and prunes, sultanas and apricots have a good variety of nutrients. All fruits are rich in carbohydrates.

Sources of ideas

Fruits in the widest sense – including pulses, nuts, grains and those like tomatoes that we eat as vegetables – can supply all the nutrients you need. Look in vegetarian cookbooks or on some of the websites listed on page 30 for ways of making fruits part of your diet. Ideas include eating fruit as toppings with cereal, in salads and as juices to drink.

Food bites

Colourful fruit

The colours of fruits highlight the health and disease-fighting chemicals they contain.

Red (chemicals against cancer, diabetes, memory loss) Cranberries, strawberries, tomatoes, raspberries, cherries, pink grapefruits, guavas

Orange-yellow (chemicals against heart diseases) Apricots, oranges, pears, pineapples, peaches, canteloupe melons, lemons, mangoes, yellow grapefruits

Green (chemicals for healthy eyes, bones and teeth) Kiwis, honeydew melons, green grapes, green apples, avocados, figs

Blue-violet (chemicals against cancer, diabetes, memory loss) Prunes, raisins, plums, blueberries, blackberries, black grapes.

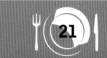

Using what you eat

Foods and drinks that enter your body must be broken down to release their nutrients and energy. This is the process of digestion. It starts in your mouth, continues in your stomach and small intestine and ends at your anus. It involves digestive juices from your salivary glands, pancreas and small intestine. The juices contain chemicals known as enzymes that break down proteins, fats and carbohydrates into small units.

▼ Fruits are easily digested, quickly releasing their energy. This makes them great for snacks.

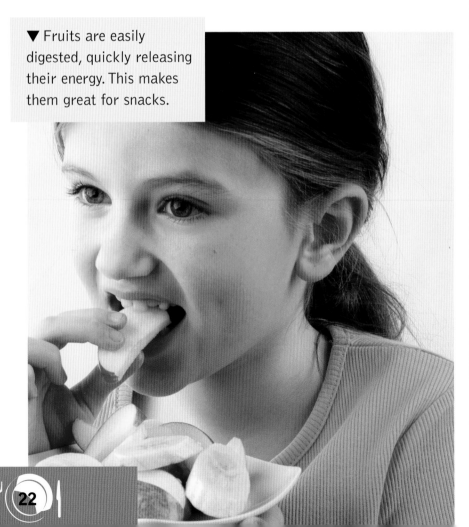

Nutrition facts

Vitamin profiles

Vitamin A gives you healthy eyes, blood and bones. Peaches, melons, dried apricots and prunes are good sources.

B vitamins prevent heart disease and cancer. Many fruits contain very little.

Vitamin C fights infections. You will find it in blackcurrants, strawberries and citrus fruits. Dried fruits do not contain any vitamin C.

Vitamin D gives you healthy bones and helps to prevent cancer. Fruits lack vitamin D.

Vitamin E prevents cell damage. Fruits contain very little of this.

Vitamin K gives you healthy blood and bones. There is little in fruits.

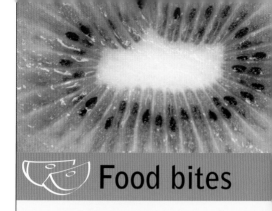

The story of glucose

Fruits are mostly carbohydrates. Enzymes in saliva start to break them down into medium-sized sugars. Little else happens until these sugars enter the small intestine. There they are broken down into glucose, the smallest and simplest sugar in the body. The whole process takes several hours.

Digested fruit material, including the vitamins and minerals, passes out of your intestine and into your bloodstream. From there it passes to your liver. Here, one of three things happens. Some glucose goes straight away to provide energy to cells and tissues that make up your body. Glucose may be stored in the liver and your muscles for use as energy a little later. Any extra glucose is changed into fats and stored for use as energy much later on. If these fats are not used up, you put on body weight.

Fruit material left over is mostly fibre that aids digestion. This is pushed out of your body as faeces.

Food bites

The easy way out

If the waste your body is getting rid of is too hard or soft, you can regulate it with fruit. As many mothers of babies know, bananas and apple sauce will make stools (poo) firmer, while dried fruit – especially prunes – will loosen it. If it works for babies, it is safe for you to try.

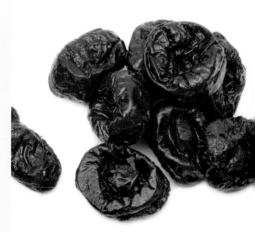

▲ Prunes help digestion. They can be eaten on their own, stewed or with cereals.

Health facts

The digestive system

The liver and pancreas produce chemicals that help digestion. Broken-down food is processed by the liver.

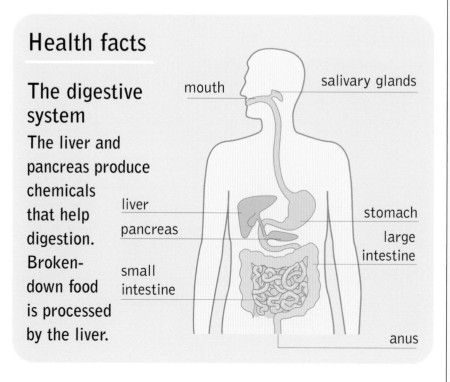

mouth — salivary glands — liver — pancreas — small intestine — stomach — large intestine — anus

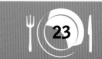

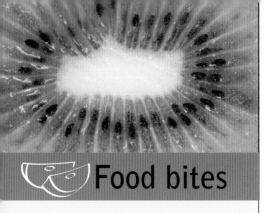

A day's worth of energy – a fruit-rich diet

kcal	meals
	breakfast
210	2 pancakes with 1 sliced peach
130	1 glass pineapple juice
	lunch
360	peanut butter and strawberry jam on multigrain bread
110	1 apple
102	1 glass semi-skimmed milk
80	1 bowl green, leafy salad with oil and vinegar
	snack
163	1 scoop low-fat cottage cheese
36	1/2 cup tinned mandarin oranges
105	1 banana
	dinner
262	small roast turkey breast
52	1 scoop cranberry sauce
22	1/2 cup steamed green beans
145	1 baked potato in jacket
271	1 piece blueberry pie
2,048	**GRAND TOTAL**

Energy balance

Although fruits are rich in carbohydrates, many of them are made up largely of water. Compared to meat, fish, eggs, grains and pulses, fruits have fewer kilocalories for the same weight. This means you can eat more of them without putting on weight. The number of kilocalories you need depends on your age, gender and how active you are. The figures on page 25 give you an idea of how much energy you need.

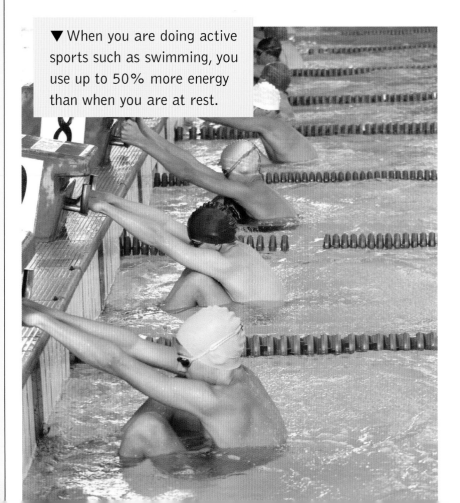

▼ When you are doing active sports such as swimming, you use up to 50% more energy than when you are at rest.

Nutrition facts

Using up energy

One large pear will give you enough energy for one of these activities:

8 minutes of running on the spot

11 minutes of walking up stairs

14 minutes of wrestling, judo or karate

16 minutes of cross-country skiing

27 minutes of basketball

28 minutes of cycling or horseback riding

36 minutes of laughing

53 minutes of walking at 3 km/hr

Fruits and sport

Fruits such as bananas release their energy slowly. They are good to eat before and after sport, exercise or training. Citrus fruits are refreshing to eat during and after long sporting activities. Whatever activity you do, match your energy intake with what your body needs.

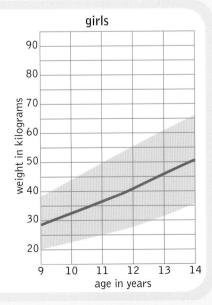

Food bites

Daily energy needs

children aged 7-10
  about 2,000 kcal

girls aged 11-14
  about 2,200 kcal

boys aged 11-14
  about 2,500 kcal

To compare the kilocalories in various foods and drinks, look at the nutrition details on food labels or on the Internet.

1 kcal = 4.2 kJ

Health facts

Body weight

Look at the correct graph. For your age, check that your weight lies close to the average – shown by the red line. If it does not, ask advice from a doctor or dietician to help you adjust your energy intake.

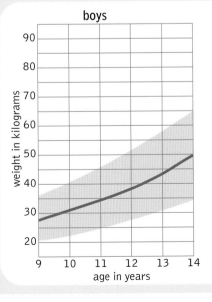

Choosing fruit to eat

Your family probably buys and eats fruits that are familiar. By not trying new fruits, you are missing out on some interesting and unusual tastes and textures. You may choose fruits based on cost or if they are produced in an environment-friendly way. Fruits grown locally are usually cheaper to buy than those grown far away. Less common fruits are also expensive.

The climate where you live and the seasons can also influence what fruits you can buy. In many places, fresh fruits are more plentiful in the summer and autumn. Religious and cultural traditions may make your selection of foods a little different from your friends'.

Nutrition facts

Sugar content

All of the following are types of sugars. When reading fruit product labels for ingredients, add the amounts of these listed to learn the true content of sugar. Brown sugar, corn sweetener, corn syrup, dextrose, fructose, fruit juice concentrate, glucose, honey, lactose, maltose, mannitol, maple syrup, molasses, raw sugar, sorbitol, sucrose, sugar, syrup, table sugar.

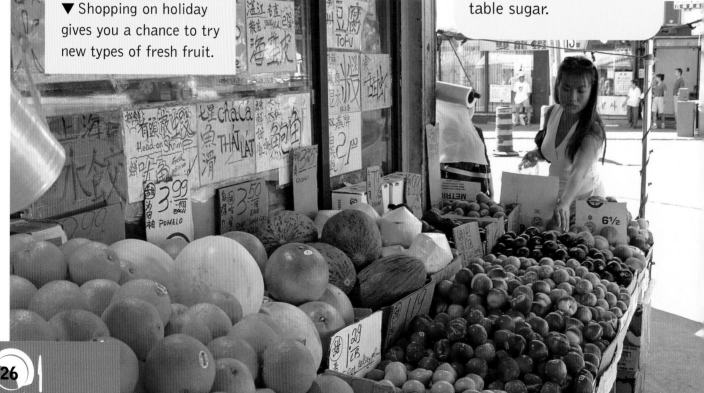

▼ Shopping on holiday gives you a chance to try new types of fresh fruit.

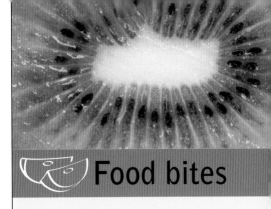

Ripening

Eat as much fresh fruit as you can. Buy it free of bruises and blemishes and eat it when it is ripe for best flavour and texture. Once harvested, fruit will continue to ripen, so any fruit you buy under-ripe will last for a few days or perhaps a week. To slow down ripening, keep fruit in a refrigerator. To speed up ripening, put fruits such as bananas, avocados and canteloupe melons in a brown paper bag.

How much fruit and sugar

With packaged fruit – bagged, tinned or frozen – read the food labels carefully. Just because the word 'fruit' appears on a package does not mean that a meaningful amount of fruit is present. Most labels do not tell you the percentage of fruit inside, but the ingredients list may give you a good idea. Usually, ingredients are listed in order, from the largest amounts to the smallest. But be careful. Sugar takes many forms and can be listed several times with different names.

▼ See-through packaging allows you to check the quality of fruits before you buy them.

Food bites

Fruit juice

When buying juice, choose 100% fruit juice, not a drink or blend filled with artificial flavours, colouring and sweeteners. Cranberry juice is an exception because it is too sour to drink without added sweetener.

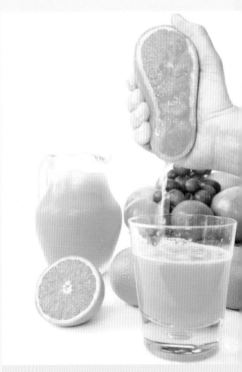

▲ Squeeze fresh oranges to make your own tasty juice.

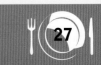

Cooking safety

Here are some rules you should follow when cooking and following recipes.

- ask an adult for permission to cook and for help in handling anything sharp or hot
- wash your hands before you begin
- after handling raw meat, wash your hands, cooking tools and surfaces with hot, soapy water
- wash fruits and vegetables before using
- use pot holders or oven gloves when handling something hot
- keep saucepan handles turned towards the back of the stove
- open saucepan lids away from you to avoid burning your face with steam
- avoid loose long sleeves, or roll them up
- keep your fingers and hair out of the way when using appliances
- never plug in appliances with wet hands

Projects

Here are some ideas for things you can do related to fruit and diet. Discover the variety of fruits that are available. Record what you are eating now and see how you can introduce more fruits into a balanced diet.

Action 1

Supermarket detective

- How many different kinds of fresh fruits can you find in your local supermarket?
- Write down the price of the same weight of five different common fruits. Compare the price of the same weight of five more unusual fruits. Is there a clear difference in price? Can you think why?
- Look at the labels to find which countries the fruits came from. Do some countries seem to produce more fruits than others and, if so, of which types of fruits?
- Take a look at the tinned, frozen and dried food sections in the supermarket. How many different kinds of fruits can you find?
- Now look at the ready-made foods section. How many of these have fruits listed as ingredients? How many tell you the amount of fruit inside?
- Look at the juice section. How many kinds of fruit juices are there? How many of them are 100% fruit juice?

Food tracking

Make a chart like the one shown below. For five days, every time you eat a piece of fruit, put a tick into the appropriate box or boxes. Note with an X every time you drink 100% fruit juice.

   At the end of the five days, count the number of ticks for each day. If there are any Xs noted, add 1 to the total number of ticks for that day. (Remember, fruit juice counts as only one serving, no matter how much you drink.) Write these totals in the bottom row. Now, add up how many fruits of different colours you ate during the five days. Write these totals in the right-hand column.

FRUIT COLOURS	Monday	Tuesday	Wednesday	Thursday	Friday	Total colours
green						
yellow-orange						
blue-violet						
red						
white						
TOTAL FRUITS						
Number of ticks						

- How often did you eat fruit during the week?
- What is the average number of ticks recorded each day?
- On how many days did you eat fruit of every colour?
- Which colour did you eat the most often?

Make a fruit list

What fruits do you eat now? Next time you go food shopping, see how many other fruits are available.

Are some fruits available in the shops only at certain times of the year? Can you think of any reasons why? Do more of the fruits come from the United States, Africa and the Mediterranean countries of Europe than from the rest of the world? Why do you think this is?

Discuss the different fruits you eat with your friends. Do they eat the same as you? What are your favourite fruits and what are theirs? Discuss your reasons why.

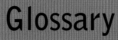

Glossary

CARBOHYDRATES
One of the three main nutrients in food. They are made of sugar molecules and mostly provide energy.

DIET
The food and drink that a person eats.

CONCENTRATE
Fruit juice with most of the water removed.

ENZYMES
Substances that help digestion and other chemical processes.

FATS
One of the three main nutrients in food. They are made of fatty acids and glycerol and mostly provide an energy store.

GRAINS
The edible seeds of grass plants.

INGREDIENTS
Individual items of food that are required to make a particular dish.

KILOCALORIES (kcal)
The units used to measure the energy in food and drink. Kilojoules (kJ) are also used.

MINERALS
Nutrients needed in small amounts for health. They include iron, calcium, phosphorus, sodium and zinc.

NUTRIENTS
Materials the body needs but cannot make itself.

OILS
Fats that are naturally liquid.

PESTICIDES
Chemicals sprayed on plants to kill other living things that may damage them or infect them.

POULTRY
Birds kept for meat and eggs, in particular chickens, turkeys and ducks. Their meat is called 'white meat' to contrast with red meat.

PRESERVATION
Ways of stopping food going bad. They include drying, freezing and packing in tins.

PROTEINS
One of the three main nutrients in food. They are made of amino acids and mostly provide building materials for the body.

RED MEAT
Meat rich in blood, such as beef, lamb, veal, pork and venison.

TROPICAL
From the region of the world between the Tropic of Cancer to the north of the Equator and the Tropic of Capricorn to the south. The climate is mostly warm or hot and moist.

VITAMINS
Nutrients needed in small quantities for health, fitness and body processes.

Websites

Here is a selection of websites that have information and activities about food, diet, health and fitness.

http://www.5aday.nhs.uk/
Information from the National Health Service on eating fruits (and vegetables).

http://www.thefruitpages.com/
All kinds of information about fruit, with activities.

http://www.tradewindsfruit.com/fruits_region_frameset.htm
Click on a country for information – and often good photographs – of the fruits that grow there. Click on "fruit database" for details of tropical fruits.

http://www.pickyourown.org/united kingdom.htm
Find a farm near you where you can pick your own fruit.

http://www.foodsubs.com/FGFruit.html
Lots of information on different kinds of fruits, including photographs and even a few recipes.

http://www.webvalley.co.uk/brogdale/home.php
A fruit catalogue that lists the 2,040 varieties of apples and 337 varieties of plums in the National Fruit Collection.

http://www.uga.edu/fruit/
An encyclopedia of the world's major fruit crops, assembled by a university horticulture professor who also accepts e-mailed questions.

http://www.eatwell.gov.uk/info/games/
The government Food Standards Agency site, with information and interactive games for children about food and health.

http://www.blubberbuster.com/height_weight.html
Allows you to calculate your Body Mass Index.

http://www.foodafactoflife.org.uk/
Educational material about food, diet and nutrients.

http://www.vegsoc.org/
Food information for vegetarians.

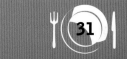